In a COVID-19 World, Become a Survivor

Other books by this author

- **Microscopic Colitis**
- **Understanding Microscopic Colitis**
- **Vitamin D and Autoimmune Disease**
- **8 Ways to Prevent Pancreatic Cancer**
- **Why Magnesium Is the Key to Long-Term Health**
- **Stroke Recovery**

In a COVID-19 World, Become a Survivor

Boost Your Immune System Now

Wayne Persky

Persky Farms

United States

First published and distributed in the United States of America by:

Persky Farms, 19242 Darrs Creek Rd, Bartlett, TX 76511-4460. Tel.: (1)254-718-1125; Fax: (1)254-527-3682. www.perskyfarms.com

Copyright: This book is protected under the US Copyright Act of 1976, as amended, and all other applicable international, federal, state, and local laws. All rights reserved. No part of this book may be reproduced by any mechanical, photographic, or electronic process, or in the form of an audio recording, nor may it be transmitted or otherwise copied for public or private use, other than the "fair use" purposes allowed by copyright law, without prior written permission of the publisher.

Disclaimer and Legal Notice: The information contained in this book is intended solely for general educational purposes, and is not intended, nor implied, to be a substitute for professional medical advice relative to any specific medical condition or question. The advice of a physician or other health care provider should always be sought for any questions regarding any medical condition. Specific diagnoses and therapies can only be provided by the reader's physician. Any use of the information in this book is at the reader's discretion. The author and the publisher specifically disclaim any and all liability arising directly or indirectly from the use or application of any information contained in this book.

Please note that much of the information in this book is based on personal experience and anecdotal evidence. Although the author and publisher have made every reasonable attempt to achieve complete accuracy of the content, they assume no responsibility for errors or omissions. If you should choose to use any of this information, use it according to your best judgment, and at your own risk. Because your particular situation will not exactly match the examples upon which this information is based, you should adjust your use of the information and recommendations to fit your own personal situation.

This book does not recommend or endorse any specific tests, products, procedures, opinions, or other information that may be mentioned anywhere in the book. This information is provided for educational purposes, and reliance on any tests, products, procedures, or opinions mentioned in the book is solely at the reader's own risk.

Any trademarks, service marks, product names, or named features are assumed to be the property of their respective owners, and are used only for reference. There is no implied endorsement when these terms are used in this book.

Copyright © Wayne Persky, 2020. All rights reserved worldwide.

ISBN 978-1-7328220-2-3

Introduction

This book contains the basic information needed to allow most people to boost their immune system, in order to improve their disease resistance, and improve their long-term health. The information discussed and the suggestions offered are based on actual published medical research that you can verify yourself from the listed references. After strengthening your immune system, you should find that you will be significantly more resistant to infections and disease, including autoimmune diseases, cancer, and viruses such as the flu, colds, and the coronaviruses.

Much of the information on vitamin D and magnesium in this book is discussed in much greater detail in some of the other books by this author, listed above. So if you would like to see additional information, the books titled Vitamin D and Autoimmune Disease and Why Magnesium Is the Key to Long-Term Health are suggested reading.

This book will help you to:

- Identify deficiencies that weaken your immune system
- Understand why these deficiencies exist
- Rate the effects these deficiencies can have on your health
- Learn how to correct these deficiencies
- Maximize your overall disease resistance
- Have fewer colds, flu, or other viruses each year
- Minimize your symptoms if you do catch a cold or virus
- Minimize COVID-19 risks for you and your family
- Enjoy better long-term health, with fewer doctor visits

How did our ancestors survive?

How Does the Body Normally Protect Itself From Disease?

The first humans evolved on this planet over a million years ago. And obviously they did it without the help of any type of health care system. Early on, the world was a dangerous place to live. It was inhabited by large predators that saw humans as just another food source. Various pathogenic bacteria were common, and most food soon spoiled, because there was no way to preserve it. Viruses were also common, and pandemics were inevitable as tribes learned to establish trade routes that allowed them to enrich their lives by trading with tribes from other areas, and eventually, other parts of the world. But the human body is an amazingly complex organism, and because most of these pathogenic threats existed before and during the time that humans evolved, the human immune system evolved to be able to deal with them.

Injuries and infections were inevitable. If one of our paleolithic ancestors became injured or sick, they couldn't go see a doctor to get a prescription for an antibiotic, or buy a disinfectant at the corner pharmacy. Their immune system had to be able to deal with it, or else they had no choice but to suffer the consequences.

In a Covid-19 World, Become a Survivor

So like every other organism that hopes to survive in this often hostile world, humans developed a very robust immune system early on. It functioned automatically, and it learned to deal with every health issue that we encountered during the many generations over which we evolved.

The true beauty of our immune system is that it evolved to take care of it's needs by using sunlight and the mineral magnesium as fuel.

Sunlight was freely available most days, and magnesium was always plentiful in the diet of early humans, because the early soil composition of most areas of the earth contained abundant reserves of magnesium. Ground water and growing plants readily absorbed magnesium. The paleo people mostly relied on hunting wild animals for their food. And since the animals absorbed the magnesium in the plants that they ate, and both the animals and our early ancestors drank magnesium-rich water, early humans always had relatively high levels of magnesium in their bodies.

And since early humans were out in the sun for most of the day, they soaked up plenty of sunlight that their bodies automatically converted into vitamin D. So the immune systems of early humans almost always provided good protection against most infections and viruses. Although people living at northern latitudes tended to run short of sunlight during the winter months,

How Does the Body Normally Protect Itself From Disease?

they avoided a vitamin D deficiency though, by eating oily fish that provided a good source of vitamin D.
And any individuals or tribes that did not have an adequate immune system were soon taken out of the gene pool by the process of natural selection. Over the millennia, occasional virus pandemics made sure that the immune systems of survivors were robust, and able to deal with the latest virus developments.

But beginning about a century ago, as more people began to leave the farm to work in factories, many of our ancestors began to get less sunlight exposure, on the average. Then during the 1950s, when air conditioning began to become popular, people began to shun the sun even more. The development of sun screen products added fuel to the fire, so that we slowly became unable to soak up enough sun exposure to allow us to maintain anywhere near the vitamin D levels that earlier generations had enjoyed.

And unfortunately, in recent years, the distractions of the now very complex world that we live in have caused most of us to overlook and ignore our primal vitamin D requirements. And today especially, with the many restrictions imposed on us because of coronavirus threats, most of us are getting even less sun exposure, and therefore less vitamin D. This appears to be the primary reason why today, so many of us are vulnerable to the worrisome health threats imposed by coronaviruses such as COVID-19. Compared with our ancient ancestors, our immune systems today are significantly compromised. And this is happening at a time when a robust immune system may well be vitally important for providing maximum disease resistance.

Why are vitamin D and magnesium so important?

What is vitamin D?

Vitamin D is a fat-soluble vitamin that is normally produced by the skin, after exposure to sunlight. The skin can utilize ultraviolet B energy in sunlight to convert a special form of cholesterol, 7-dehydrocholesterol, into vitamin D (Wacker and Holick, 2013).[1] But this process takes roughly eight hours to be completed, so if the oily residue on the skin that contains the previtamin D is washed off by soap and water too soon, some or most of the vitamin D will be lost. A few generations ago, this wasn't normally a problem, but today, most people bathe or shower more often, so they are more likely to lose some of the benefits of vitamin D generated by sunlight. And if sunscreen is used, most of the vitamin D conversion may be blocked, anyway.

Vitamin D is also available in many foods, and as a dietary supplement. Whether it's sourced from the sun, food, or a supplement, vitamin D is stored in an inert form, and it

Why are vitamin D and magnesium so important?

cannot be used by the body until it's converted by two hydroxylation processes into the active form, 1,25-dihydroxyvitamin D, also written as [1,25(OH)2D]. When your doctor orders a blood test to measure your vitamin D level, he or she is testing vitamin D that has gone through the first hydroxylation process in the liver, 25-hydroxyvitamin D, also written as [25(OH)D].

Vitamin D is critically important for proper immune system functioning.

As the National Center for Biotechnology Information (NCBI) of the United States (U. S.) government puts it (Gunville, Mourani, & Ginde, 2013):[2]

> *Vitamin D is well known for its classic role in the maintenance of bone mineral density. However, vitamin D also has an important "non-classic" influence on the body's immune system by modulating the innate and adaptive immune system, influencing the production of important endogenous antimicrobial peptides such as cathelicidin, and regulating the inflammatory cascade. Multiple epidemiological studies in adults and children have demonstrated that vitamin D deficiency is associated with increased risk and greater severity of infection, particularly of the respiratory tract. Although the exact mechanisms by which vitamin D may improve immune responses to infection continue to be evaluated, vitamin D supplementation trials of prevention and adjunct therapy for infection are underway. Given its influence on the immune system and*

inflammatory cascade, vitamin D may have an important future role in the prevention and treatment of infection.

Quite a few authorities recommend vitamin D for helping to prevent disease. But vitamin D is only part of the solution. It only helps if the user's magnesium level is adequate, because the immune system can't use any of that vitamin D until it's activated. And magnesium is required for the activation process.

What is magnesium, and why is it important for disease resistance and good health.

Physically, magnesium is a solid, gray in color. As a chemical element, it's listed on the periodic table with an atomic number of 12 and the abbreviation Mg. It's an electrolyte, which means that when it's dissolved in certain solvents, it produces an electrically conducting solution. The significance of this is that it's also electrically conducting in blood serum, which allows it to facilitate many vital chemical processes in the body.

One of the more important chemical functions that magnesium provides is to act as a cofactor to convert the inactive form of vitamin D into the active form.

This property is vital not only for our immune system functioning, but for many other chemical processes required by the body as well. Without the active form of vitamin D, our immune system cannot function as intended. As previously mentioned,

Why are vitamin D and magnesium so important?

until it's activated, vitamin D is normally stored in the form of 25-hydroxyvitamin D, also written as 25(OH)D. Whether naturally sourced from the sun or provided by an oral vitamin D supplement, vitamin D is always stored in the inactive form. But our body cannot use vitamin D in the inactive form. It has to be converted into the active form in order to be utilized. The active form of vitamin D, known as 1,25-dihydroxyvitamin D, is often written as 1,25-(OH)2D. Medical research published many decades ago proved that when magnesium supplies are inadequate, the human body is unable to use vitamin D, due to the inability to convert it into the active form. So that makes an adequate magnesium level essential for proper immune system functioning.

Uwitonze and Razzaque, (2018) did a good job of summing up the importance of magnesium for activating vitamin D in their abstract of an article they wrote that was published by the American Osteopathic Association.[3]

> *Nutrients usually act in a coordinated manner in the body. Intestinal absorption and subsequent metabolism of a particular nutrient, to a certain extent, is dependent on the availability of other nutrients. Magnesium and vitamin D are 2 essential nutrients that are necessary for the physiologic functions of various organs. Magnesium assists in the activation of vitamin D, which helps regulate calcium and phosphate homeostasis to influence the growth and maintenance of bones. All of the enzymes that metabolize vitamin D seem to require magnesium, which acts as a cofactor in the enzymatic reactions in the liver and kidneys. Deficiency in either of these nutrients*

is reported to be associated with various disorders, such as skeletal deformities, cardiovascular diseases, and metabolic syndrome. It is therefore essential to ensure that the recommended amount of magnesium is consumed to obtain the optimal benefits of vitamin D.

But the virtues of magnesium go far beyond that.

As mentioned previously, magnesium is not just another nutrient. As a vital electrolyte, magnesium assists the body in regulating our heart rate, breathing, blood pressure, temperature, and various other important functions. Our magnesium level, together with our vitamin D level, has a huge effect on our ability to heal. So blood levels of these two critical nutrients probably explain why some people are able to heal much faster than others. Published research shows that healing is severely compromised when either magnesium or vitamin D is deficient. Maintaining adequate levels is especially important for anyone who is fighting any disease or an infection. And it's vital for maintaining a good level of resistance to prevent the development of a disease or infection.

It's a fact of life that young people heal much faster than older people.

But part of the reason for this difference is due to the fact that as we age, our general ability to digest many foods decreases. Stomach acid production decreases, and our ability to produce adequate digestive enzymes to assist in digestion also slowly

Why are vitamin D and magnesium so important?

deceases. So fewer nutrients are available to us, and our ability to absorb those nutrients is also likely to diminish.

Older people are much more likely than younger people to be taking a medication. Many common medications deplete vitamin D and magnesium, and doctors don't usually adequately warn patients before writing a prescription for them. Proton pump inhibitors (PPIs), for example, deplete magnesium so aggressively that the FDA has issued a warning that for some people, a PPI treatment absolutely must be ended before those individuals will be able to restore their magnesium levels and correct their magnesium deficiency.

Furthermore, many older people have an autoimmune issue, or some other chronic disease, and many chronic issues, especially inflammatory bowel diseases (IBDs) significantly deplete the absorption of magnesium and vitamin D.

Why have most of us developed these deficiencies?

In prehistoric times, most soils contained more-than-adequate levels of magnesium.

And this was still true up until about the last century. But after centuries (thousands of years in some areas) of farming, magnesium levels in many soils have slowly become depleted as growing plants absorb the magnesium, and it's not being replaced. Prior to modern farming methods of the last few centuries, when plants took up the magnesium, they later rotted in place and the magnesium was returned to the soil. Or it was returned to the soil by the manure of the animals that ate the plants. Recently, as farming methods have become much more intensive, plants still absorb the available magnesium, but much of the magnesium is never returned to the soil. Consequently, many soils now contain far lower levels of magnesium, so that our foods contain much less magnesium than they did even just a few decades ago. We're no longer eating food that has the quality of the food that our great-grandparents ate. And our general health is beginning to reflect that sad reality.

Up until a few generations ago, drinking water was a significant source of magnesium.

In many areas, it was possible for many people to get much of their magnesium requirements from their drinking water. But since then, drinking water has been subjected to increasingly more intense filtering and chemical treatment processing, until today, most drinking water contains almost no magnesium.

Our paleo ancestors apparently were able to get most of their magnesium requirements from water. Water was the only beverage that they routinely drank. And most streams, rivers, and lakes contained water that had a relatively high magnesium level, because the water ran across rocks and soil that had a high magnesium content. It appears that up until a few generations ago, that was still generally true.

Why have most of us developed these deficiencies?

But today, drinking water supplies only a fraction of the magnesium we need.

Because of parasites, and contamination with chemicals and various pathogens, drinking untreated water has become a very risky proposition. So these days, all drinking water systems are treated by filtering and processing with chemicals so that it will meet state and federal guidelines. And even so, the water in many areas of the country often fails to meet safe guidelines. But as the water treatments become increasingly more intense, our drinking water contains progressively less magnesium. And to make sure that our personal drinking water is safe, today many households have their own water filtration systems. So most of our drinking water contains so little magnesium in many areas today, that we can reasonably assume that we're not getting enough magnesium from our drinking water to even be worth considering.

According to many authorities, the average adult needs to drink a minimum of about two liters of water per day in order to maintain good health. But in February of 2007, a researcher (Kiefer) published a study of bottled water and municipal water supplies that showed that two liters of either bottled water or the water available in most cities in the U. S., only contained about 10 to 20 percent of the recommended daily allowance (RDA) for magnesium.[4]

Clearly, we can no longer rely on our drinking water to supply the magnesium we need. Nor can we rely on food raised on magnesium-depleted soils for our magnesium requirements. Yet our generation has done little or nothing to offset and correct this problem, so it's not surprising that most people today would be magnesium deficient.

Some authorities estimate that approximately 80 % of the general population is now magnesium deficient.

And this percentage is almost surely weighted toward the older citizens in the population. Yet the medical community continues to generally ignore the serious implications of this increasing problem.

So it's not surprising that the medical profession continues to describe new diseases from time to time And why should we be surprised to discover that food sensitivities and allergies are increasing? After all, the immune system cannot function properly when vitamin D is deficient, or adequate magnesium is not available to activate it.

Diagnoses of type 2 diabetes are rapidly increasing. It's becoming a very common disease. And sure enough, there is published medical research that proves that magnesium deficiency is closely associated with type 2 diabetes (Takaya,Higashino, & Kobayashi, 2004).[5] In that research article the authors concluded that magnesium is essential not only for glucose metabolism, but also for insulin signaling. Inadequate magnesium can induce insulin resistance. They showed that both hypertension and type 2 diabetes involve low cellular magnesium levels.

Why have most of us developed these deficiencies?

Furthermore, this means that magnesium and insulin are co-dependent. Insulin's primary function in the body is to transport nutrients from the bloodstream to the cells of the body where those nutrients are needed. This implies that as insulin resistance increases, magnesium may not be properly transported to cells, making this a potentially self-perpetuating problem as the body's cells become even more starved for magnesium. Furthermore, magnesium deficiency can lead to reduced insulin production by the pancreas, further depleting insulin. Once someone becomes caught in this spiral it becomes increasingly difficult for them to utilize the magnesium in their diet, resulting in an increased risk of insulin resistance. When either magnesium or insulin levels become inadequate, the risk of developing diabetes or a condition known as pre-diabetes increases significantly. But proper supplementation with magnesium can treat and resolve pre-diabetes if it's done before pre-diabetes becomes diabetes and requires medical treatment.

Ever wonder why the Mediterranean Diet is so popular, and so effective for reducing the risk of heart disease, stroke, diabetes, and various other health problems? It contains a relatively high amount of magnesium. Likewise, vegetarian or vegan diets typically offer similar health benefits because they, too, normally contain larger amounts of magnesium than most other common Western diets.

Because most people living today are magnesium deficient, that suggests that those who do not have a magnesium deficiency should have a lower risk of most common health issues. King, Mainous, Geesey, & Woolson (2005) have not only shown that

In a Covid-19 World, Become a Survivor

most Americans are magnesium deficient, but they proved that adequate magnesium intake will lower the C-reactive protein (CRP) level of those individuals.[6] As you probably are aware, doctors commonly test patient's CRP levels to help assess their risk of cardiovascular disease. Higher CRP levels correlate with a higher risk of cardiovascular disease.

To illustrate how damaging a magnesium deficiency can be, Mazur et al.. (2007) proved that only a few days of magnesium deficiency for laboratory rats was sufficient to cause chronic inflammation.[7] But the researchers also proved that the rats' inflammation level could be decreased by increasing the magnesium levels of those rats.

Therefore we have proof that a magnesium deficiency promotes inflammation in the body. It's well known that most diseases, including autoimmune diseases, and even cancer, are caused by chronic inflammation. This implies that allowing ourselves to become magnesium deficient, may be putting our general health at risk. A magnesium deficiency clearly increases our risk of developing exactly the assorted diseases that we would prefer to avoid. The risk of developing certain diseases is significantly influenced by our gene pool. And if any autoimmune diseases develop, that increases the odds that additional autoimmune diseases will develop, because many autoimmune diseases deplete vitamin D and magnesium, so the process can become a vicious cycle .

Why do these problems continue to be mostly ignored by the medical community?

For the most part, the medical community overlooks and generally ignores the increasing problem with chronic magnesium deficiency among the general public. Probably the main reason why physicians fail to recognize this issue is because the so-called "normal" range for an acceptable magnesium test result level appears to be too low. Medical practitioners continue to ignore the issue despite the fact that researchers pointed this out many years ago (Liebscher and Liebscher, 2004).[8]

According to Dr, Carolyn Dean, a published expert on magnesium deficiency who has written a number of books on the subject, argues that because the original "normal" range used data that was based on a cohort in which approximately 80 % of the subjects were magnesium deficient, the normal range is skewed toward the low end.[9] Therefore test results within the so-called "normal" range may actually indicate a magnesium deficiency.

The magnesium test traditionally ordered by doctors is a poor choice.

The type of test that's ordered, determines whether the results will be useful for determining the patients magnesium status.

In a Covid-19 World, Become a Survivor

Doctors typically order a serum magnesium test, which reports the amount of magnesium available at the moment in the patient's blood.

But this test is only useful in an Emergency Room setting where a healthcare team is searching for the reasons why a patient is having issues serious enough to prompt them to come to the Emergency Room seeking medical help. Since magnesium is a vital electrolyte, it's blood level is automatically regulated by the body within a relatively narrow "normal" range. If the level is too high, the body discards some of the magnesium to bring the level back down to within the normal range. If it's too low, the body draws on reserves stored in muscle cells.

So the serum test will only show a deficiency if all the reserves are almost completely depleted, which can eventually led to a life-threatening risk of cardiac arrest. This makes the test ideally suited for an Emergency Room situation. As The National Institutes of Health points out, less than one percent of the body's total supply of magnesium is available in blood serum, making it a rather poor choice for most testing purposes.

So their magnesium reserve level is actually the test result that most patients normally need to know.

Therefore, when a patient goes to his or her doctor for routine (none-emergency) visits, the magnesium test ordered by the doctor should be one that tests cellular reserves. Though several types of such tests have been developed, the only one that's

Why do these problems continue to be mostly ignored by the medical community?

commonly (and economically) available is the red blood cell (RBC) magnesium test. Doctors will usually agree to order this test when the patient requests it (in lieu of the serum test), and the results will be much, much, more accurate and useful for determining the patients actual magnesium sufficiency or insufficiency.

But due to the fact that the original "normal" range was based on data collected from a cohort that was about 80 % magnesium deficient, the desired result should be in the upper part of the normal range used by most labs. Many labs today use a normal range of approximately 3.8–6.4 mg/dL According to Dr Carolyn Dean, a test result of 6.0 mg/dL or above is desirable, especially for someone who has all the symptoms of a magnesium deficiency, such as insomnia, migraines, atrial fibrillation, leg cramps, or muscle twitching.

Have you ever been awakened by leg or foot cramps, while sleeping? A deficiency of any electrolyte can cause the problem, but in most cases, those late-night or early-morning cramps are caused by a magnesium deficiency. It happens because as the magnesium from your last meal that's in circulation in your bloodstream is slowly used up, your body begins to withdraw magnesium previously stored in your muscles to replace it. The leg muscles are good reservoirs for storing magnesium, since they're large enough to provide a significant amount of storage. But when your magnesium reserves begin to run low, the result is leg and foot cramps.

In a Covid-19 World, Become a Survivor

After your first meal of the day, the cycle is restarted as the magnesium in your food boosts your blood level enough that some of the excess magnesium will be sent to your muscles to be stored until needed. But the cramps are clear evidence that your reserves of one or more electrolytes are too low, implying that you need to be ingesting more magnesium, or whatever electrolyte is deficient. In the vast majority of cases, magnesium deficiency is the problem.

Severe magnesium deficiency can lead to a dangerous situation. It can cause cardiac issues, even including cardiac arrest, because the heart is a muscle, and it will begin to cramp up if it runs too low on magnesium. Despite the fact that the mainstream medical community continues to mostly ignore the widespread magnesium deficiency problem among the general population, published medical research has been available to them for many years showing the health advantages of correcting magnesium deficiencies.

Research clearly shows that simply correcting magnesium deficiencies can eliminate many serious health problems, including heart disease and hypertension (Touyz, 2004).[10] And resolving magnesium deficiencies often eliminates or attenuates many less serious conditions that tend to be troublesome or even debilitating for some people. As an example, magnesium deficiency is so prevalent among fibromyalgia patients that many experts believe that fibromyalgia may be just another symptom of magnesium deficiency (Deans, 2012, September 11).[11] There are even published articles showing that magnesium can be used to treat fibromyalgia (Engen, et al., 2015).[12]

Why do these problems continue to be mostly ignored by the medical community?

More people are becoming health conscious when they shop for food these days.

They carefully read labels and choose foods with fewer unhealthy ingredients. Allergies have become more common during the last generation or two, so many shoppers read labels to make sure that the products they buy are safe for themselves and other family members. Awareness of the increasing prevalence of hypertension, diabetes, autoimmune diseases, and cancer, has inspired many people to avoid foods with numerous chemical preservatives listed on the label.

But what if the nutritional value of many of our foods is not as good as we are led to believe it is?

By law, the labels on processed foods must contain certain basic nutritional information. And the government has published lists of official RDAs for all common foods. But are we capable of actually absorbing all those nutrients? Many factors can compromise our ability to absorb certain nutrients. Just because the nutrients are in the food, doesn't mean that we'll be able to absorb them. Nutritional data are often determined under generally perfect conditions, in a laboratory setting. Obviously, we won't be eating those foods under perfect conditions. And our meals are certainly not consumed under laboratory conditions.

Many of the nutrients in food are lost during the cooking process.

More than a few of those nutrients are discarded with the liquids in which the foods are cooked. So they're diminished before we even eat the food. And our own personal ability to absorb the nutrients that remain in the food after it's cooked can be very different from that of a government bureaucrat's definition of an "average" individual. Our ability to absorb nutrients depends on our genetics, our age, our gut bacteria profile, our general health , our activity level, any digestive system issues that we might have, and possibly other conditions. And then there are certain foods that inhibit the absorption of certain nutrients in our diet, or deplete certain nutrients already in our bodies.. Our paleo ancestors never ate such foods. But we consume them every day. And of course it's highly unlikely that the government's RDA guidelines accurately allow for the effects of foods that inhibit nutrient absorption or deplete nutrients. Since we're interested in boosting our immune system, we'll focus on foods that deplete magnesium or vitamin D.

More people are becoming health conscious when they shop for food these days.

Many medications are known to deplete magnesium.

In fact, many of the most commonly-prescribed medications severely deplete magnesium. Corticosteroids, certain antibiotics, antacids, contraceptives, cardiovascular drugs, diuretics, and as previously mentioned, protein pump inhibitors (PPIs) are some of the worst. Usually, medications such as these won't completely block the absorption of magnesium, but some of them severely limit absorption.

And conversely, while they are reducing the absorption of magnesium, the process of depleting the magnesium often also limits the efficacy of the medication. For example, certain antibiotics may become only marginally effective in the presence of significant magnesium levels in the bloodstream. In some cases, the effect may be significant enough to prevent the antibiotic from doing it's intended job. Bactrim and Ciprofloxacin are examples of antibiotic that fall into this category.

Probably the worst class of medication known to deplete magnesium is the PPIs. After extended use, they tend to deplete magnesium so severely that the FDA issued a special warning to specifically address this issue. Here's a quote from that warning (FDA Drug Safety Communication: (2011, March 2).[13]

> *[3-2-2011] The U.S. Food and Drug Administration (FDA) is informing the public that prescription proton pump inhibitor*

> *(PPI) drugs may cause low serum magnesium levels (hypomagnesemia) if taken for prolonged periods of time (in most cases, longer than one year). In approximately one-quarter of the cases reviewed, magnesium supplementation alone did not improve low serum magnesium levels and the PPI had to be discontinued.*

Note the last sentence in that quote. If you read the label on PPIs, their FDA label only specifies that they should be used for a few weeks. Yet once people start using them, PPIs often create a dependency, (because if a PPI is stopped, the symptoms return even worse than they were, originally) so that many people tend to use PPIs for very long periods . . . even indefinitely. Then eventually, the severe magnesium deficiency begins to cause additional health problems.

Have the official government-issued RDAs become outdated?

The RDAs were established decades ago. Why would we believe that some average number derived from a selected cohort of people would be representative for our particular needs? People come in a wide variety of sizes and shapes, and in general, our own nutritional needs are unique to our genetics, weight, metabolism, physical activity, environment, general health status, any health issues, and probably many other factors, in some cases. How could some average number possibly be accurate for every one of us? And even if those RDAs were accurate several decades ago, how accurate are they today? There have been a lot of changes during that time. There are many experts who

More people are becoming health conscious when they shop for food these days.

disagree with some of the more important RDA listings, such as vitamin D, and they advocate higher vitamin D intake for disease prevention (Giovannucci, (2007, April 26).[14]

Rickets is a disease caused by a severe vitamin D deficiency, and it was a major problem before the 1940s. But after the benefits of vitamin D were discovered, in the early 1940s, most developed countries were able to wipe out rickets by requiring food processors to enrich certain foods with vitamin D.

The problem is, those recommendations haven't been updated to keep up with current research, and we're apparently still using those vitamin D RDA levels established back in the pre World War II era. And as might be expected, those vitamin D levels are barely adequate for preventing rickets. Diseases such as cancer and viruses, and most other health problems, are tougher to handle, and they require that the immune system have higher blood levels of vitamin D available.

It's been well-established by medical research, that an adequate vitamin D level is essential for preventing common chronic diseases such as autoimmune diseases, bone metabolic disorders, cardiovascular diseases, diabetes, neuropsychiatric disorders, and tumors (Wang, et al., 2017).[15]

We live in a different world today.
Especially now that we have all the health risks imposed by the coronaviruses hanging over us. And from all indications, based on the ways that viruses can quickly mutate to stay ahead of

effective vaccine developments, we may be living with a cyclic coronavirus threat for decades into the future. Today we're dealing with derivatives of the SARS-CoV-2 coronavirus strain. How this threat will evolve in the future, we can't even make a decent guess, but one thing is certain — it's not likely to just fade away on it's own. It will take many years of dedicated work to finally end the ever-present risk of infection. And as world population levels continue to increase, additional coronaviruses will almost surely become a problem at some point in the future, and we, or our descendants, will be forced to contend with them.

Vitamin D sufficiency is critical for resistance against the coronaviruses.

If there's one truly valuable finding coming out of all the research being done on COVID-19, it's that the vitamin D level of Covid-19 patients is critically important for preventing severe symptoms and minimizing the mortality risk. So we have the information we need to protect ourselves from the worst risks attributed to this family of diseases. We have to keep our immune system in optimum condition so that it can protect us. If we become infected, unless we have certain severe underlying conditions, our immune system should be able to prevent any severe symptoms from any virus. Even if we have underlying conditions, a robust immune system should help to minimize our symptoms. The value of vitamin D against COVID-19 is well documented by recent medical research (Kaufman, et al., 2020).[16] In that study of test results for over 190,000 people, the data showed that those who had a serum vitamin D level of 55 ng/mL

More people are becoming health conscious when they shop for food these days.

(138 nmol/l), or higher, were less than half as likely to have a positive COVID-19 test result as those who had a vitamin D serum level below 20 ng/mL (50 nmol/l).

Researchers at Northwestern University collected data from hospitals and clinics all over the world, and analyzed it. Data from China, France, Germany, Italy, Iran, South Korea, Spain, Switzerland, the United Kingdom (UK) and the United States were included (Northwestern University, May 7, 2020).[17] Not surprisingly, they found that reduced patient vitamin D levels were consistently associated with higher mortality rates from COVID-19.

Some authorities had speculated earlier that vitamin D might contribute to the risk of cytokine storms, which are known to be the cause of many mortalities from COVID-19. But researchers proved that speculation to be incorrect, In fact, the researches found that the data was so consistent between vitamin D deficiencies and an increased mortality risk, that they concluded that not only does vitamin D strengthen our innate immune systems, but it's also protective against immune systems becoming dangerously overactive, thereby helping to prevent cytokine storms (Daneshkhah, et al., Preprint posted 2020, April 30).[18]

Yet another group of medical researchers have shown that in their study, having a vitamin D deficiency almost doubled the risk of developing COVID-19, compared with those who did not have a vitamin D deficiency (Meltzer, et al., 2020, September 3).[19] In this study, a vitamin D deficiency was defined as having a

In a Covid-19 World, Become a Survivor

serum vitamin D level below 20 ng/mL (50 nmol/l). As we might expect, the research team hypothesized that vitamin D supplementation might be helpful for lowering the risk of developing COVID-19.

Another recently-published study among COVID-19 patients, show that those who have a serum vitamin D level in the sufficient range have a significantly reduced risk of mortality, or severe symptoms, compared with those who have a serum vitamin D level that's considered to be deficient (Melville, 2020, September 30).[20] That study also demonstrated how higher serum levels of vitamin D were associated with improved outcomes for COVID-19 patients, due to a reduced risk of cytokine storms.

A study of 200 COVID-19 patients in a Spanish hospital found that over 80 % of them had serum vitamin D levels that were in the deficient range(The Endocrine Society, 2020, October 27).[21] Importantly, they discovered that the men in the study had lower serum vitamin D levels than the women. This appears to be a possible contributing factor to explain why men generally have a higher mortality risk from COVID-19, than women.

The study also noted that COVID-19 patients who had lower serum vitamin D levels, also had generally higher levels of certain laboratory markers of inflammation, such as ferritin and D-dimer. While it's also a measure of iron status, when increased levels of ferritin are found in overweight and obese patients it can be used as an inflammation marker. And D-dimer is a small fragment of protein left in the blood after a blood clot

More people are becoming health conscious when they shop for food these days.

is dissipated by fibrinolysis. This suggests that patients who have higher serum vitamin D levels appear to have fewer issues with the blood-clotting problems that are so often caused by COVID-19, and often lead to severe symptoms, or a fatal outcome.

Researchers in Italy have published the results of a much more important study that illustrates the fact that a low serum level of vitamin D is an independent risk factor associated with the development of more severe COVID-19 symptoms that typically require admission into an intensive care unit, and significantly raises the risk of a fatal outcome (Busko, 2020. September 17).[22] In the study, done on patients from a Milan hospital, there were 103 symptomatic patients, 52 with positive tests but mild symptoms, and 206 healthy controls. The patients who had to be admitted into the hospital had the lowest serum vitamin D levels, at a mean of 18.2 ng/mL (45.5 nmol/l). The patients who had mild symptoms had a mean serum vitamin D level of 30.3 ng/mL (75.8 nmol/l), while those in the control group had a mean serum vitamin D level of 25.4 ng/mL (63.5 nmol/l).

Among the patients with mild symptoms, 79 % were taking a vitamin D supplement. But only 30 % of those who were hospitalized were taking a vitamin D supplement. Those who were hospitalized also were slightly older, and they were more likely to have a preexisting health problem. 54 of the patients in the hospitalized group required treatment in an ICU, and 19 of them died, The hospitalized patients who did not require treatment in an ICU, had a mean serum vitamin D level of 22.4 ng/mL (56 nmol/l), while those who required ICU treatment had a mean serum vitamin D level of 14.4 ng/mL (36 nmol/l). Those who died had a mean serum vitamin D level of 13.2 ng/mL (33 nmol/l).

As a result of all this compelling research data, the medical community is finally recommending that everyone should be using supplemental vitamin D to help reduce the number of COVID-19 new infections, and to limit the risk of severe symptoms in those patients who do develop the disease. Hopefully, this will help to significantly reduce the number of fatalities resulting from this disease.

Hyperglycemia is associated with mortality risk for COVID-19 patients.

Hyperglycemia was found be a predictor of death or other severe outcome in a Spanish study, regardless of diabetes status.[23] More than 11,000 patients in 109 Spanish hospitals were included in the study, and those with an abnormally-high blood glucose level at hospital admission were more than twice as likely to die from the disease than those with normal glucose levels (41.4 % vs 15.7 %). They were also more likely to need a ventilator or require admission into an intensive care unit (ICU).

This wasn't part of that study, but please note that a chronic magnesium deficiency often leads to an elevated blood glucose level (hyperglycemia).[24]

And what are the current medical recommendations regarding magnesium, with respect to COVID-19?

Not surprisingly, there are none. The medical community continues to fail to recognize the critical importance of magnesium for supporting our immune systems, thereby ignoring the critical effect that may have on our disease resistance. They embrace the benefits of vitamin D for helping to prevent and minimize dangerous complications that often result from COVID-19. But they fail to point out that vitamin D supplementation can be ineffective if an individual has a magnesium deficiency. The reduction in efficacy depends on the extent of the deficiency, and other factors specific to each individual's situation.

Because (as previously noted), about 80 % of the general population is magnesium deficient, It follows that about 80 % of the population will have compromised disease resistance that will make them more vulnerable, especially to aggressive diseases such as the coronaviruses.

Remember the study mentioned a few pages back, regarding the patients in a Spanish hospital? The researchers discovered that over 80 % of them had a vitamin D deficiency. Note that this percentage matches the generally estimated approximate percentage of the general population that's currently magnesium deficient. Hmmm. Coincidence? Probably not. In the world of science, there's a reason for everything. Actual events may seem chaotic at times, but they're driven by the rule of cause and effect. Nothing happens by coincidence, although that's a popular misconception (Beck, 2016, February 23).[25]

Look at the data from the Italian study that was mentioned next. According to the study, 79 % of the patients who had mild symptoms were taking a vitamin D supplement, and they did not require hospitalization. Only 30 % of the hospitalized patients were taking a vitamin D supplement, and we have no information on how much vitamin D they were taking — it may have been very little. If most of those hospitalized patients had not been taking a vitamin D supplement, there's a very good chance that they had not been taking a magnesium supplement, either.

People who don't take vitamin D, usually don't take any other vitamins or minerals, except maybe a multivitamin. Therefore, it's rather unlikely that they would be taking a magnesium supplement. So it appears that there's a very good chance that some or all of the patients who were vitamin D deficient (in both studies), may have also been magnesium deficient, and their magnesium deficiency may have been the primary reason why they were vitamin D deficient in the first place. After all, a magnesium deficiency will limit the body's ability to absorb vitamin D from food (Dai, et al., 2018).[26]

The biggest problem with multivitamins is that they normally don't contain enough of any of the important vitamins to even

And what are the current medical recommendations regarding magnesium, with respect to COVID-19?

come close to resolving a deficiency of any of those vitamins. And the types of vitamins included are always in the cheapest forms that the manufacturers can find.

Magnesium, for example, is virtually always in the form of magnesium oxide, despite published research showing that human digestive systems are only capable of absorbing approximately 3 or 4 percent of the elemental magnesium in magnesium oxide. Since multivitamins contain only very low amounts of magnesium oxide, to begin with, the magnesium in multivitamins typically provides no significant benefits for anyone taking those products.

We've already noted how current government agency official RDAs are only adequate for preventing rickets. Epidemiological evidence indicates that higher serum vitamin D levels are capable of decreasing the risk of developing many (maybe all) diseases, including cancer and cardiovascular disease.

But look at how the medical researchers approach this issue.

The results of a medical research trial comparing the use of vitamin D supplements with a placebo were published online in 2018, and in the prestigious New England Journal of Medicine in 2019. You may have heard about the results. The researchers concluded that vitamin D showed no benefit in preventing cancer or cardiovascular disease (Manson, et al., 2019).[27]

In a Covid-19 World, Become a Survivor

But let's just analyze the way that study was set up, to see what we can discover. Looking at the "Methods" section in the published research article, the researchers supplemented the daily diets of the subjects with either 2,000 IU of vitamin D, or a placebo. The trial design and oversight states these specific requirements for participants:

> *Eligible participants had no history of cancer (except nonmelanoma skin cancer) or cardiovascular disease at trial entry, and they were required to agree to limit the use of vitamin D from all supplemental sources, including multivitamins, to 800 IU per day and to complete a 3-month placebo run-in phase.*

So to guarantee that none of the participants in the study might have a higher serum vitamin D level, the participants were required to begin the trial with their vitamin D intake at a minimum rate. That is, their vitamin D intake was limited to only what they could derive from their regular diet, or their diet plus a vitamin D supplement of 800 IU or less. This guaranteed that their serum vitamin D level would be relatively low. Then for the trial, they were either given 2,000 IU of vitamin D daily, or a placebo. It sort of appears that this trial was designed to fail, as though the researchers were trying to prove a predetermined agenda — namely, that supplementing with vitamin D has no benefit.

Previously-published research had proven that 2,000 IU of vitamin D per day, is not even enough to maintain vitamin D

And what are the current medical recommendations regarding magnesium, with respect to COVID-19?

sufficiency at or above 30 ng/mL (75 nmol/l) (Sadat-Ali, Al-Anii, Al-Turki, AlBadran, and AlShammari, (2018).[28]
So in order to prove any cancer or cardiovascular benefits from supplementing with vitamin D, Manson, et al. would have had to use much higher vitamin D supplementation rates. How could they logically expect to prove any cancer or cardiovascular benefits from a vitamin D supplementation rate so low that it had already been proven to be inadequate to even maintain the status quo?

Not only was the Manson trial a waste of money (because of the low vitamin D supplementation rate), but it did patients all over the world a grave disservice by incorrectly convincing doctors everywhere that higher vitamin D supplementation rates are not beneficial. And now a high percentage of the world's population is trying to defend itself against a coronavirus pandemic, with a weakened immune system, because their doctors have misinformed them about supplementing with vitamin D (and failed to point out the importance of magnesium). Many people will die as a result of COVID-19, because they were misled for years about optimum vitamin D levels.

What the researchers proved is technically correct — supplementing with vitamin D at such a low rate will show no benefit. But the misleading way in which the study was structured, was either incompetent, or unscrupulous.

Many health experts outside the mainstream medical community disagree with the official medical position regarding the use of these supplements.

Because of research studies such as the ones cited as references in this book, many health authorities believe that significantly higher levels of vitamin D are beneficial for reducing the risks associated with many health threats, including COVID-19. They recommend serum vitamin D levels well above the 20 ng/mL (50 nmol/l) level considered by the medical community to be sufficient. The GrassRootsHealth Nutrient Research Institute, for example, recommends that everyone should maintain a serum vitamin D level of 40–60 ng/mL (100–150 nmol/l).[29] They even publish tables that show the relative reduction in risk levels for certain health issues using their own interpretation of various medical studies, including the Manson, et al., study.[30]

Supporting your immune system, so that it can defend you against most health issues, including COVID-19, and any other coronaviruses that may develop in the future from SARS-CoV-2, is not rocket science. It simply requires using the common sense approach of making sure that your immune system has all the fuel it needs to function at optimum levels. And basically, that means keeping your serum vitamin D level well above existing official recommendations of 20 ng/mL (50 nmol/l). If maximizing disease resistance is your goal, then you need to do your

Many health experts outside the mainstream medical community disagree with the official medical position regarding the use of these supplements.

best to maintain a vitamin D level in the 40–60 ng/mL (100–150 nmol/l) range. Taking too much vitamin D carries little risk, because as long as one's serum vitamin D level remains below 100 ng/mL (250 nmol/l), overdose symptoms are very unlikely.

A level above about 150 ng/mL (375 nmol/l), will cause many individuals to have overdose symptoms. Overdose symptoms include digestive upset, diarrhea, and possibly other issues. Statistics show that most overdose cases on record have resulted from situations where individuals took 40,000 IU or more of vitamin D for months. If you're going to take daily doses of 10,000 IU or more, be sure to have your serum vitamin D level checked every few months or more frequently, to make sure that you don't overdose. It's better to keep supplementation rates in the 5,000–7,000 IU range, and check blood levels of vitamin D every 3–6 months, so that you can fine tune your daily dose to meet your needs, because some people need more vitamin D than others.

You're probably wondering how to determine whether you need a magnesium supplement in the first place. Of course, according to statistics, there's automatically about an 80% chance that you do. If you have leg or foot cramps during the night, you probably do. If you're low on energy, and fatigue easily, you probably do. If you want to be sure, ask your doctor to order an RBC magnesium test for you, and carefully examine the results while ignoring the lab recommendations. If your result is up in the range that Dr. Carolyn Dean recommends (as discussed back on page 17), then you're fine and your present magnesium intake is

In a Covid-19 World, Become a Survivor

ideal. But if your result is below that desired range then a magnesium supplement would almost surely benefit you.

If you happen to have compromised kidney function, check with your doctor before starting to take a magnesium supplement. Since magnesium is an electrolyte, it's blood level is regulated by the body so that it stays within what's called a normal range. Any excess magnesium above that range is removed from the blood by the kidneys, so if you have reduced kidney function, taking a magnesium supplement that exceeds your needs could cause excessive work for your kidneys. And if blood levels of magnesium should get too high, the elevated level could cause cardiovascular issues, thus the reason for checking with your doctor before starting to take a magnesium supplement.

Otherwise, if your kidneys are working normally, you should have no trouble when taking a magnesium supplement. If you're magnesium deficient, taking between 200 and 400 mg daily should work satisfactorily, depending on your needs, for getting your magnesium reserves built back up to a satisfactory level. After your magnesium reserves are restored, the supplement dose should be reduced, so that it matches the normal magnesium RDA shortfall in your diet. The RDA for men is 400–420 mg, and the RDA for women is 300–320 mg. Since blood levels of magnesium are closely regulated by the body, it's best to divide your daily dose between meals, because if the total dose is all taken at the same time, much of it may be wasted by the kidneys as it's removed in order to keep the blood level within the normal range.

Many health experts outside the mainstream medical community disagree with the official medical position regarding the use of these supplements.

There are many types of magnesium supplements to choose from. The best type is probably magnesium glycinate (chelated magnesium). It's well-absorbed by the body, and it's the least likely form to cause diarrhea. The worst type is probably magnesium oxide. Human digestive systems can only absorb about 3 or 4 % of magnesium oxide, which means that the rest will remain in the intestines, where it may cause diarrhea.

Our paleo ancestors were bigger and much stronger than we are today.

The archaeological records clearly show this to be the case. They not only survived, but thrived in many varied environments that were often challenging, and dangerous. They controlled bacteria and infections with their immune system, rather than antibiotics. They didn't drink coffee, or alcohol, and since they had no medications, their magnesium and vitamin D levels were never at risk of becoming depleted for unnatural reasons. They absorbed plenty of vitamin D from being out in the sun all day, and their food and drinking water contained plenty of magnesium, in those days. Tribes that lived in northern climates, where sun exposure was greatly reduced, and drinking water was often derived from melted snow, kept their immune systems robust by eating oily fish and seals that were rich in vitamin D and magnesium.

Our species will probably never again be as big and strong as our paleo ancestors. But we can regain some of that lost advan-

In a Covid-19 World, Become a Survivor

tage by taking vitamin D and magnesium supplements that will help us to keep our immune systems as robust as possible. If we will just do that, we've minimized, and maybe even eliminated the risk of severe COVID-19 complications and most other common health risks.

Of course, preexisting conditions can cause complications in any case. And those who have suppressed immune systems due to medical intervention (such as those taking immune system suppressants) will also have an increased risk. But that risk will be significantly diminished if they maintain good vitamin D and magnesium levels. Bear in mind that most of the underlying conditions that increase the risk of adverse events due to COVID-19 will not be a problem in the first place, if we always maintain our vitamin D and magnesium at good levels. Published research shows that magnesium treats prediabetes and hypertension. And it prevents type 2 diabetes.

Good vitamin D and magnesium levels eliminate most immune system problems (other than taking a drug designed to suppress your immune system). If you want to further insure that your immune system will be able to protect you from most viruses and adverse coronavirus events, taking a daily vitamin C, and a zinc/copper supplement will eliminate a deficiency of these important elements, if you should happen to have a deficiency of any of them. The actual amount of zinc and copper in the body is not nearly as important as the ratio of the two. Most authorities agree that the long-term balance should be approximately 15 to 1. In other words, a zinc/copper supplement that contains

Many health experts outside the mainstream medical community disagree with the official medical position regarding the use of these supplements.

about 50 mg of zinc, and 2 or 3 mg of copper, is ideal for helping to keep your immune system as fit as a fiddle.

Even after good vaccines become available, and assuming that our immune system is in optimum condition, it will still behoove us to take all the normal precautions to try to prevent being exposed to COVID-19 (or any other mutation derived from the family of coronaviruses), especially if we're among the older, more vulnerable generation. But unlike relying on a vaccine, which may or may not work, we can take comfort in knowing that if we should be accidentally exposed to the virus, we've done everything we can to boost our immune system, so that it should protect us to the greatest extent possible. There are no guarantees in life, but keeping our immune systems functioning as well as possible, is the closest we can come to guaranteeing that we will be survivors of this, and the next pandemic.

About the Author

Wayne Persky BSME

Wayne Persky was born, grew up, and currently lives in Central Texas. He is a graduate of the University of Texas at Austin, College of Engineering, with postgraduate studies in mechanical engineering, mathematics, and computer science. He has teaching experience in engineering, and business experience in farming and agribusiness. He has 20 years of experience researching published medical research articles to discover novel ways to resolve health issues that are inadequately treated by mainstream medicine.

Microscopic colitis (MC) is an inflammatory bowel disease more widespread than Chron's disease, yet the most popular medical treatment used by doctors results in an 85 % relapse rate. He promotes treating MC by diet changes, with a better than 95 % success rate. Over 15 years ago he founded and continues to administrate an online MC discussion and support board. In 2015 he founded the Microscopic Colitis Foundation, and he continues to serve as it's president and as a contributing author to the Foundation's Newsletter. He lives on a farm in Central Texas, where he continues to do research and write.

Contact Details:

In a Covid-19 World, Become a Survivor

Wayne Persky can be contacted at:
Persky Farms
19242 Darrs Creek Rd
Bartlett, TX 76511
USA

Tel: 1(254)718-1125
Tel: 1(254)527-3682

Email: wayne@perskyfarms.com
Email: wayne@microscopiccolitisfoundation.org
Email: wayne@waynepersky.com

For information and support regarding microscopic colitis, visit:

https://www.microscopiccolitisfoundation.org/
To view or participate in the Microscopic Colitis Discussion and Support Forum, go to:

https://www.perskyfarms.com/phpBB/index.php

1. Wacker, M., and Holick, M. F. (2013). Sunlight and vitamin D. *Dermato Endocrinology*, Retrieved from https://www.ncbi.nlm.nih.gov/pmc/articles/PMC3897598/

2. Gunville, C. F., Mourani, P. M., & Ginde, A. A. (2013). The role of vitamin D in prevention and treatment of infection. *Inflammation & Allergy - Drug Targets*, 12(4) 239–245. Retrieved from https://www.ncbi.nlm.nih.gov/pmc/articles/PMC3756814/

3. Uwitonze, A. M., and Razzaque, M. S. (2018). Role of magnesium in vitamin D activation and function. *The Journal of the American Osteopathic Association*, 118(3), 181–189. Retrieved from https://jaoa.org/article.aspx?articleid=2673882

4. Kiefer, D. (2007, February). Is your bottled water killing you? *Life Extension Magazine*, Retrieved from http://www.lifeextension.com/magazine/2007/2/report_water/Page-01

5. Takaya J., Higashino H., & Kobayashi, Y. (2004). Intracellular magnesium and insulin resistance. *Magnesium Research*, 17(2), 126–136. Retrieved from https://pubmed.ncbi.nlm.nih.gov/15319146/

6. King, D. E., Mainous, A. G. 3rd, Geesey, M. E., & Woolson, R. F. (2005). Dietary magnesium and C-reactive protein levels. *The Journal of The American College of Nutrition*, 24(3), 166-171. Retrieved from https://www.ncbi.nlm.nih.gov/pubmed/15930481

7 Mazur, A., Maier, J. A., Rock, E., Gueux, E., Nowacki, W., & Rayssiguier, Y. (2007). Magnesium and the inflammatory response: potential physiopathological implications. *Archives of Biochemistry and Biophysics*, 458(1), 48–56. Retrieved from https://www.ncbi.nlm.nih.gov/pubmed/16712775

8 Liebscher D. H., & Liebscher, D. E. (2004). About the misdiagnosis of magnesium deficiency. *The Journal of the American College of Nutrition*, 23(6), 730S–731S. Retrieved from https://www.ncbi.nlm.nih.gov/pubmed/15637222

9 Dean, C. (2015, October 20). Why test for magnesium? [Web log message]. Retrieved from https://drcarolyndean.com/2015/10/why-test-for-magnesium/

10 Touyz, R. M. (2004). Magnesium in clinical medicine. Frontiers in Bioscience, 1(9), 1278–1293. Retrieved from

11 Deans, E. (2012, September 11). Is fibromyalgia due to a mineral deficiency? Psychology Today. Retrieved from https://www.psychologytoday.com/blog/evolutionary-psychiatry/201209/is-fibromyalgia-due-mineral-deficiency

12 Engen, D. J., McAllister, S. J., Whipple, M. O., Cha, S. S., Dion, L. J., Vincent, A., . . . Wahner-Roedler, D. L. (2015). Effects of transdermal magnesium chloride on quality of life for patients with fibromyalgia: a feasibility study. Journal of Integrative Medicine, 13(5), 306–313. Retrieved from https://www.ncbi.nlm.nih.gov/pubmed/26343101

13 FDA Drug Safety Communication: (2011, March 2). Low magnesium levels can be associated with long-term use of proton pump inhibitor drugs (PPIs). U.S. Food and Drug Administration [Web log message]. Retrieved from
http://www.fda.gov/Drugs/DrugSafety/ucm245011.htm

14 Giovannucci, E. (2007, April 26). Ask the expert: Vitamin D and chronic disease. Retrieved from https://www.hsph.harvard.edu/nutritionsource/2007/04/26/ask-the-expert-vitamin-d-and-chronic-disease/

15 Wang, H., Chen, W., Li, D., Yin, X., Zhang, X., Olsen, N. . . . Zheng, S. G. (2017). Vitamin D and Chronic Diseases. Retrieved from https://www.ncbi.nlm.nih.gov/pmc/articles/PMC5440113/

16 Kaufman, H. W., Niles, J.K., Kroll, M. H., Bi, C., & Holick, M. F. (2020). SARS-CoV-2 positivity rates associated with circulating 25-hydroxyvitamin D levels. Retrieved from https://journals.plos.org/plosone/article?id=10.1371/journal.pone.0239252

17 Northwestern University. (May 7, 2020). Vitamin D levels appear to play role in COVID-19 mortality rates. Retrieved from

18 Daneshkhah, A., Agrawal, V., Eshein, A., Subramanian, H., Roy, H. K., & Backman, V. (Preprint posted April 30, 2020). The possible role of vitamin D in suppressing cytokine storm and associated mortality in COVID-19 patients. Retrieved from

https://www.medrxiv.org/content/10.1101/2020.04.08.20058578v3

19 Meltzer, D. O., Best, T. J., Zhang, H., Vokes, T., Arora, V. A., & Solway, J. (2020, September 3). Association of vitamin D status and other clinical characteristics with COVID-19 test results. Retrieved from https://jamanetwork.com/journals/jamanetworkopen/fullarticle/2770157

20 Melville, N. A. (2020, September 30). More evidence that vitamin D sufficiency equals less severe COVID-19. Retrieved from https://www.medscape.com/viewarticle/938303?src=mkm_covid_update_200930_mscpedit_&uac=95382HN&impID=2595919&faf=1

21 The Endocrine Society. (2020, October 27). Over 80 percent of COVID-19 patients have vitamin D deficiency, study finds. Retrieved from https://www.sciencedaily.com/releases/2020/10/201027092216.htm

22 Busko, M. (2020. September 17). Low vitamin D in COVID-19 predicts ICU admission, poor survival. Retrieved from https://www.medscape.com/viewarticle/937567

23 Tucker, M. E, (2020 November 30). Blood glucose on admission predicts COVID-19 severity in all. Retrieved from https://www.medscape.com/viewarticle/941716?src=mkm_covid_update_201130_MSCPEDIT&uac=95382HN&impID=2707601&faf=1

24 Fulop, T. (2020, October 30). What is the role of hypomagnesemia in the etiology of diabetes? Retrieved from https://www.medscape.com/answers/2038394-35970/what-is-the-role-of-hypomagnesemia-in-the-etiology-of-diabetes

25 Beck, J. (2016, February 23). Coincidences and the meaning of life. Retrieved from https://www.theatlantic.com/science/archive/2016/02/the-true-meaning-of-coincidences/463164/

26 Dai, Q., Zhu, X., Manson, J. E., Song, Y., Li, X., Franke, A. A., . . . Shrubsole, M. J. (2018). Magnesium status and supplementation influence vitamin D status and metabolism: Results from a randomized trial. *The American Journal of Clinical Nutrition.* 108(6), pp 1249–1258. Retrieved from https://academic.oup.com/ajcn/article/108/6/1249/5239886

27 Manson, J. E., Cook, N. R., Lee, I-M., Christen, W., Bassuk, S. S., Mora, S. . . . Buring, J. E. (2019). Vitamin D supplements and prevention of cancer and cardiovascular disease. The New England Journal of Medicine, 380, p 33-44 Retrieved from https://www.nejm.org/doi/full/10.1056/nejmoa1809944

28 Sadat-Ali, M., Al-Anii, F. M., Al-Turki, H. A., AlBadran, A. A., & AlShammari, S. M. (2018). Journal of Bone Metabolism, 25(3), pp 161–164. Retrieved from https://www.ncbi.nlm.nih.gov/pmc/articles/PMC6135651/

29 The GrassrootsHealth Nutrient Research Institute. (nd). Current Recommendations are Too Low. Retrieved from https://www.grassrootshealth.net/blog/current-recommendations-low/

30 GrassrootsHealth Nutrient Research Institute. (2018). Risk Reduction with Vitamin D and Omega-3: VITAL Trial Results (2018). Retrieved from http://grassrootshealth.net/wp-content/uploads/2018/11/VITAL-Results_D-O3-Benefits.pdf

www.ingramcontent.com/pod-product-compliance
Lightning Source LLC
Chambersburg PA
CBHW071126030426
42336CB00013BA/2219